AF894134

After the Center for Weight Loss Success Jump Start

Dr. Clark's
CENTER FOR
WEIGHT LOSS
SUCCESS

After the Jump Start

Congratulations on completing Dr. Clark's 2-Week Jump Start Program!!

You should be very proud of yourself and your commitment to losing weight and improving your health. We realize that the past two weeks might not have been easy but you have demonstrated great control and your 5-25 pound weight loss should feel great! Who doesn't enjoy more energy and better fitting clothes? Congratulations again!

Now that you have lost weight and "jump started" your path to improved health, don't stop now. You are 14 days closer to your goal and we want to help you meet or exceed your ultimate longer-term health goal(s) as well. We see success every day and we are thrilled to have you as a part of our weight loss family.

So where do you go from here? **First** of all, celebrate you! Celebrate in moderation if it includes food or better yet, celebrate your success with something non-food related like a new piece of clothing or manicure/pedicure if that suits your fancy. It's all about you!

Second, make a plan for your continued success and a manageable way of eating that fits with you and your lifestyle. To help you with this, we have developed this "After the Jump Start" guide. The information here can be followed indefinitely and customized to your likes/dislikes. Remember…it needs to be something YOU can live with for life. The plan includes two options – one that continues use of protein shakes for 3 meals/day and the other includes an easy-to-follow meal plan that includes per meal guidelines/choice along with delicious recipes that are simple to prepare.

Now to the details of your *After the Jump Start* plan:

You have already demonstrated your dedication to success. Now it is time to figure out how to continue your healthier way of eating without feeling deprived long-term rather than thinking of this as a "diet" that is short term.

You have a couple of options after completion of Dr. Clark's 14-day Jump Start Program.

1. You can continue to have a shake for breakfast, lunch, and snack and then eat a healthy dinner (Mini Jump Start Plan at CFWLS*) *or*
2. You can eliminate the protein shakes for some of your meals and transition to an entire menu of healthy meals/snacks. You know yourself best and you understand if the predictability and simplicity of a shake will be better or not for you long-term. Both are outlined on the next pages.

*(Jump Start and Mini Jump Start may be alternated for continued quick results).

Option 1 - Mini Jump Start Plan

This is a food and protein supplementation diet consisting of approximately 1100 - 1200 calories depending on food choices selected. It is ideal for individuals who wish to "accelerate" their weight loss and get on the right track with a flexible healthy eating plan. The afternoon snack may be taken mid-morning instead.

Breakfast (200 calories): 1 Weight & Inches shake*

Lunch (200 calories): 1 Weight & Inches shake

Afternoon Snack (200 calories): 1 Weight & Inches shake

Main Meal (approx. 500-600 calories):

Include protein, salad, and vegetable.

Protein (approx. 200-250 calories):

1 serving daily (approx. cooked weight) from the following with all skin, bone, visible fat removed and use a cooking method that does not add fat.

5 oz ground beef (lean 10%), lean steak, veal, or pork

6 oz chicken or turkey

6 oz venison or ham

6-8 oz white fish, shell fish, or canned fish (must be water packed or rinsed)

Salad (approx 50 calories):

2 cups lettuce or other leafy greens

1 cup vegetables (celery, tomato, cucumber, etc.)

AND

Low calorie dressing (25 calorie limit) **OR** vinegar, salt, lemon juice and other desired spices

Vegetables (approx. 50-100 calories):

Choose 1 cup cooked broccoli, spinach, beets, asparagus, carrots, green beans or cauliflower

Water/Beverages:

Try to drink ***at least*** 8 cups (64oz) of water each day.

You can drink other beverages as long as they are calorie-free (less than 5 calories per serving) and caffeine-free. Suggestions for these types of beverages include decaf coffee and tea, decaf diet soda, Crystal Light, diet seltzer or diet mineral water, and herbal teas. Remember, caffeine acts as a diuretic and causes you to lose water from your body. If you must have caffeine please limit to one serving per day.

Journaling:

We recommend that all of our patients begin journaling your food and fluid intake as well as daily exercise using your journal. We will want you to continue journaling throughout your weight loss journey to help you become more conscious of your food selections and intake – and to track your success!

To get the most out of this plan, Dr. Clark recommends these 4 additional vitamins/ nutrients:

- Complete Multi-Vitamin (2 tabs/day)
- Essential Fatty Acids (EFA's) (2 gel capsules 2 times/day)
- Activated B-Complex (1-2 capsules/day)
- Magnesium/Potassium Aspartate (1 twice/day)

You may also want to consider adding B-Complex injections to help prevent fatigue, commonly associated with calorie restricted diet plans.

*The Weight & Inches shake comes in chocolate and vanilla flavors (7 per box). They can be purchased at the CFWLS Nutritional Store, 645 J. Clyde Morris Blvd., Newport News, VA or online at www.cfwls.com (the cost is less than $3.00/meal) – you can't beat that!

Option 2 - Your Easy-To-Follow Meal Planning Guide

There are a couple of things for you to consider as you get started. Please don't get overwhelmed – I promise we will keep this as simple as possible for you.

First, what to count (don't glaze over here this is important). If you count one thing, count your carbohydrate intake. You should try to keep that intake below 50 grams/day. If you count two things, count your carbohydrate and protein intake. We can help you determine your specific protein need but in the meantime, try to keep it to twice your amount of carbohydrate (so around 100 grams/day).

Second, plan your meals ahead of time and record what you plan to eat. This can be done easily on our portable App (search for CFWLS or Center for Weight Loss Success in your app store) ***or*** you can plan your meals and record what you eat on the forms included on the next two pages or online at www.myfitnesspal.com or www.fitday.com.

Third, use the awesome " Effective Carbohydrate Content" document included with this plan. It should be with you at all times as you plan your meals.

Fourth, when you plan your meals and snacks keep the guidelines and recipes in this book in mind.

Fifth, Enjoy this journey towards a healthier you. As Dr. Clark says: " Life is what we do minute to minute and day to day...It's your life, make it a healthy one!"

You are worth it, and we are here to help. If you have any questions, contact us at success@cfwls.com or 757-873-1880.

My Daily Food Journal

Date ______________________

Time	Place	Food/Drink	Calories	Protein	Eff. Carb	*	**	Comments

Date ______________________ * Excessive Behavior **Hunger Scale (1-5)

Time	Place	Food/Drink	Calories	Protein	Eff. Carb	*	**	Comments

Weekly Menu Planner

Week of ______________

	Breakfast	Lunch	Dinner
Monday			
Tuesday			
Wednesday			
Thursday			
Friday			
Saturday			
Sunday			

Notes:

Shopping List

Breakfast Ideas

Breakfast is an essential part of your daily diet.

The Weight and Inches shakes are perfect but here are 7 other good choices!

1	**Weight & Inches shake**
2	1 cup 2% cottage cheese
3	2 eggs with turkey bacon
4	Proti hot chocolate & a cheese stick
5	CFWLS oatmeal & cappuccino
6	Low-carb English muffin with egg and slice of Canadian bacon
7	2 egg omelet with cheese
8	Leaner Living shake blended with 4-5 frozen strawberries

Tasty Snacks On The Go

Snack Possibilities

Snack	Portion	Protein	Carb
Sunflower Seeds	1 oz.	5	4
Walnuts	1 oz.	4	5
Macadamia Nuts	1 oz.	3	4
Peanuts	1 oz.	7	5
Pork Rinds	1 oz.	17	0
Lean Meat Slices	1 oz.	7	0-1
String Cheese	1 oz.	6	1
Meat/cheese/cracker	½ oz each on 2 crackers	7	4
Homemade peanut butter crackers	1 T/2 crackers	4	5
Hard-cooked Egg	1 large	6	0.6
Cottage Cheese	¼ cup	7	2
Apple/Cheddar Slices	¼ apple/1 oz.	7	6
Jerky	1 oz.	7	1
Sandwich (light bread, 1 oz. meat)	½	7	7

Quick & Easy Lunches

Keep your lunches easy but vary the choices
from day to day so that you don't get bored or feel deprived.

1	**Salad greens with 3-4 oz grilled chicken & colorful veggies**
2	Cup of plain Greek yogurt mixed with CFWLS pudding & shake
3	Chicken salad in low-carb pita
4	Grilled chicken nuggets and side salad
5	Weight & Inches Shake
6	Low-carb wrap with hummus and turkey, baby spinach & tomato
7	Bowl of chili with sprinkle of cheese

Simple Dinner Recipes

garlic and lemon tilapia

Difficulty: Easy

prep time
10 minutes

cook time
15 minutes

serves
2

Serve with:
Side Salad
Steamed broccoli

things you need:

2 4 oz. tilapia filets, thawed & patted dry

2 cloves garlic, minced

1 tbsp. butter

1 tbsp. lemon juice

3/4 tbsp. chopped parsley

Preheat oven to 400 degrees. Melt butter in saucepan and saute garlic for 1 minute. Add lemon juice and remove from heat. Place fish in a 8" square baking dish sprayed with cooking spray. Season with salt & pepper to taste. Pour lemon mixture over fish, sprinkle with parsley. Bake for 15 minutes or until flaky.

Nutritional Info for Tilapia: (per serving)

Calories 158

Protein 24g

Effective Carbohydrates 0g

Fat 6g

bacon & swiss chicken

Difficulty: Easy

prep time
20 minutes

cook time
45 minutes

serves
2

Serve with:

Spinach salad with mandarin oranges and slivered almonds

things you need:

2 6 oz. boneless, skinless chicken breasts

4 strips of bacon, cut in half

1/2 small onion, sliced

4 oz. sliced mushrooms

2 slices swiss cheese

1/2 tsp. seasoned salt

Preheat oven to 350 degrees. Place chicken in a 8" square baking dish and sprinkle with salt. Bake chicken for 40 minutes or until cooked. Cook bacon in large skillet over medium heat until crisp; place on paper towels to drain. Saute onions and mushrooms in bacon drippings. When chicken is cooked, top with bacon, onion, mushrooms, and Swiss cheese. Return to oven until cheese melts.

Nutritional Info for Chicken: (per serving)

Calories 364

Protein 38g

Effective Carbohydrates 2g

Fat 22g

southwest salmon

Difficulty: Easy

<u>prep time</u>
5 minutes
<u>cook time</u>
10 minutes

serves
2

Serve with:

Roasted brussel sprouts sprinkled dusted with cayenne pepper & sea salt

things you need:

2 6 oz. salmon filets, patted dry

1/2 can Rotel tomatoes with lime & cilantro

1/4 tsp. salt

1/8 tsp. pepper

Red pepper flakes

1/4 cup light mayonnaise

Season salmon with salt & pepper. Combine tomatoes and mayonnaise and coat both sides of filet with mixture.

Preheat a large skillet over medium heat. Place salmon and any remaining mixture in skillet and cover. Cook for 3-5 minutes on each side or until fish flakes easily.

Nutritional Info for Salmon: (per serving)

Calories 433

Protein 36g

Effective Carbohydrates 6g

Fat 25g

gorgonzola pork chops

Difficulty: Easy

<u>prep time</u>

5 minutes

<u>cook time</u>

15 minutes

serves

2

Serve with:

Wedge of baby romaine with creamy dressing

things you need:

2 butterflied pork chops

2 tbls. Italian dressing

1/8 tsp. cayenne pepper

1 roma tomato, sliced

1/4 cup crumbled gorgonzola cheese

Preheat oven broiler.

Combine salad dressing and cayenne pepper in small bowl. Brush mixture on both sides of pork chops.

Place pork chops on broiler pan and place 3-4 inches under heat for 4-5 minutes, flip and allow to broil another 4-5 minutes or until done.

Top with tomato slices and sprinkle with cheese.

Nutritional Info: (per serving)

Calories 276

Protein 38g

Effective Carbohydrates 3g

Fat 13g

italian soup

Difficulty: Easy

prep time

5 minutes

cook time

35 minutes

serves

2

Serve with:

Tomato slices with fresh mozzarella and basil, drizzled with balsamic vinegar

things you need:

10 oz Italian turkey sausage

2 cloves garlic, minced

2 cups beef broth

½ can Italian-style stewed tomatoes, undrained

½ can great Northern beans, rinsed & drained

1 zucchini, cubed

1 cup torn spinach leaves

Brown sausage with garlic in soup pot. Cut sausage into small pieces. Stir in broth and tomatoes. Season with salt and pepper to taste. Reduce heat, cover and simmer for 15 minutes. Stir in beans and zucchini. Cover; simmer another 15 minutes or until zucchini is tender. Remove from heat. Add spinach and stir until spinach is wilted.

Nutritional Info: (per serving)

Calories 320

Protein 35g

Effective Carbohydrates 15g

Fat 11g

citrus steak

Difficulty: Easy

prep time
5 minutes (day prior)

serves
2

cook time
15 minutes

Serve with:
Side salad with tomato & avocado

things you need:

2 6 oz. sirloin steaks

1 clove garlic, minced

1/2 tsp. ginger

2 oranges, juiced

Make X cross cuts on surface of steak on both sides and place in shallow dish with lid. Cut & squeeze 1 orange into small bowl. Mix with garlic and ginger; pour over meat. Marinate in refrigerator overnight.

Heat oven to broil. Broil steaks to desired doneness. Slice steak; transfer to serving dish. Cut open; squeeze second orange over meat just before serving.

Nutritional Info: (per serving)

Calories 400

Protein 37g

Effective Carbohydrates 13g

Fat 24g

mediterranean steak strips with Proti fusilli pasta

Difficulty: Easy

<u>prep time</u>

5 minutes

<u>cook time</u>

20 minutes

serves

2

Serve with:

Small side salad (this is a large dish!)

things you need:

8 oz. lean steak

1 tbls. olive oil

1/2 tsp. salt

1/2 tsp. pepper

1 clove garlic, minced

1/2 cup tomato sauce

1 tbls. Italian dressing

2 packages Proti fusilli pasta*

Shredded Parmesan cheese

*Available at the CFWLS Nutrition Store

Nutritional Info: (per serving with pasta)

Calories 480

Protein 45g

Effective Carbohydrates 12g

Fat 27g

Cut steak into thin strips. Heat oil in skillet over medium-high heat.

Combine garlic, salt and pepper. Place steak in skillet; pour tomato sauce and Italian dressing over strips. Sprinkle dry ingredients on top; mix together.

Cook steak, covered, until steak is done as desired.

Meanwhile, cook pasta to desired tenderness. Serve steak and sauce over pasta and sprinkle with parmesan cheese.

The following “Effective Carbohydrate Content” of common foods is a tool to help you count carbohydrate amounts while on a low carbohydrate diet. Low carbohydrate diets in conjunction with caloric restriction can enhance your weight loss and the breakdown of fatty tissue.

The theory behind aggressive low carbohydrate diets is that you can force your body into using ketones as an important energy source instead of relying on glucose (**ALL** carbohydrates are eventually converted to glucose). Your fatty tissue is broken down into tiny molecules called ketones and these ketones are subsequently used as an energy source.

The effective carbohydrate content is the total carbohydrate in a certain portion of food **minus** the fiber content. The fiber portion of a carbohydrate is generally not absorbed well (and therefore does **not** affect your blood sugars) and subsequently your insulin levels. Effective carbohydrate content is **NOT** equivalent to **Net Carbs** as seen on many packages.

The columns are broken down into 5 gm effective carbohydrate content units (from 5-25). You can decide how large a portion of a particular food will be allowed depending on the amount of carbohydrate you are allowed for that day. For example, if you are trying to keep your total carbohydrate count at 50 gm/day (200 cal), you can pick any combination of foods from the appropriate columns that total 50 gms (remember to take in to consideration the carbohydrates in any supplements you are using).

For 50 gm total carbohydrate/day – you could have:

- 10 five gram portions OR
- 5 ten gram portions OR
- 1 twenty gram portion, 2 ten gram portions, and 2 five gram OR
- Any other combination that totals 50 grams

Unlimited generally means that the additional carbohydrate is negligible compared to normal amounts which can be eaten.

Effective Carbohydrate Content of Fruits

FOOD	5 Grams	10 Grams	15 Grams	20 Grams	25 Grams
Apple-raw	¼ medium	½ medium	¾ medium	1 medium	1¼ medium
Apple-cooked	¼ cup	½ cup	¾ cup	1 cup	1¼ cups
Applesauce-Unsweetened	⅛ cup	¼ cup	½ cup	¾ cup	1 cup
Apricots-raw	1½ medium	3 medium	4 medium	5 medium	7 medium
Apricots-canned	4 halves	8 halves	12 halves	18 halves	20 halves
Avocado	¾ medium	1 medium	2 medium	2½ medium	3 medium
Banana-raw	-	⅓ medium	½ medium	⅔ medium	1 medium
Blackberries-raw	½ cup	¾ cup	1¼ cups	1½ cups	2 cups
Blueberries-raw	⅓ cup	½ cup	¾ cup	1 cup	1½ cups
Boysenberries-frozen	¼ cup	½ cup	1 cup	1¼ cups	1½ cups
Cantaloupe-raw	½ cup	¾ cup	1 cup	1¾ cups	2 cups
Cherries					
Sour, canned	¼ cup	½ cup	¾ cup	1 cup	1¼ cups
Sweet, raw	5 whole	10 whole	15 whole	20 whole	25 whole
Sweet, canned	-	¼ cup	½ cup	⅔ cup	¾ cup
Crabapples-raw	-	¼ cup	½ cup	¾ cup	1 cup
Cranberries-raw	⅓ cup	¾ cup	1 cup	1½ cups	2 cups
Cranberry sauce-Jellied	2 tsp	1 Tbsp	2 Tbsp	-	-
Currants-raw, Black	½ cup	¾ cup	1 cup	1½ cups	2 cups
Dates-dried, whole	-	1 whole	2 whole	3 whole	4 whole
Figs					
Raw, whole	½ medium	1 medium	1½ medium	2 medium	2½ medium
Dried, whole	-	-	1 whole	1½ whole	2 whole
Fruit cocktail					
Canned, water	¼ cup	½ cup	¾ cup	1 cup	1¼ cup
Canned, juice	-	⅓ cup	½ cup	½ cup	¾ cup
Grapefruit					
Raw	¼ whole	½ whole	¾ whole	1 whole	1½ whole
Canned, juice	¼ cup	⅓ cup	⅔ cup	¾ cup	1 cup
Grapes-seedless	⅓ cup	½ cup	1 cup	1⅓ cups	1½ cups
Guava-raw	½ medium	1 medium	1½ medium	2 medium	2½ medium

* Values for fruits are for unsweetened fruits, and fruits canned in WATER unless otherwise noted.

Effective Carbohydrate Content of Fruits

Food	5 Grams	10 Grams	15 Grams	20 Grams	25 Grams
Honeydew-raw	¼ cup	½ cup	1 cup	1¼ cups	1½ cups
Kiwifruit-raw	½ medium	1 medium	1½ medium	2 medium	2½ medium
Lemon-raw	1 medium	2 medium	3 medium	4 medium	5 medium
Lime-raw	½ medium	1 medium	2 medium	-	-
Mandarin orange-juice packed	-	⅓ cup	½ cup	¾ cup	1 cup
Mango-raw	-	¼ cup	½ cup	⅔ cup	¾ cup
Nectarine-raw	-	½ medium	1 medium	1½ medium	2 medium
Orange-raw	½ medium	¾ medium	1 medium	1½ medium	2 medium
Papaya-raw	-	¼ medium	½ medium	¾ medium	1 medium
Passionfruit-raw, purple	1 medium	2 medium	3 medium	5 medium	6 medium
Peach					
Raw	½ medium	1 medium	1½ medium	2 medium	3 medium
Canned, water	⅓ cup	¾ cup	1 cup	1⅓ cups	1¾ cups
Dried, halves	-	1 half	1½ halves	2 halves	3 halves
Pear					
Raw	¼ medium	½ medium	¾ medium	1 medium	1¼ medium
Canned, water	¼ cup	½ cup	¾ cup	1 cup	1¼ cups
Dried, halves	-	½ of a half	1 half	1½ halves	2 halves
Asian	¼ medium	¾ medium	1 medium	1½ medium	2 medium
Persimmon-raw	-	1 medium	1½ medium	2 medium	3 medium
Pineapple					
Raw	¼ cup	½ cup	¾ cup	1 cup	1½ cups
Canned, juice	-	¼ cup	⅓ cup	½ cup	⅔ cup
Plum-raw	½ medium	1 medium	1½ medium	2 medium	3 medium
Pomegranate-raw	-	¼ medium	½ medium	¾ medium	1 medium
Prunes-dried	1 whole	2 whole	3 whole	4 whole	5 whole
Quince	-	½ medium	1 medium	1½ medium	1¾ medium
Raisins	-	-	⅛ cup	⅛ cup	¼ cup
Raspberries-raw	½ cup	1 cup	1¾ cup	2 cups	3 cups
Strawberries					
Raw	¾ cup	1½ cups	2 cups	3 cups	4 cups
Frozen, unsweet	⅓ cup	½ cup	1½ cups	1½ cups	2 cups
Tangerine-raw	½ medium	1 medium	1½ medium	2 medium	2½ medium
Watermelon-raw	½ cup	¾ cup	1 cup	1½ cups	2 cups

Effective Carbohydrate Content of Breads, Cereals, and Grains

Food	5 Grams	10 Grams	15 Grams	20 Grams	25 Grams
Bagel	-	-	½ medium	½ medium	1 small
Biscuit					
Small (¾ oz)	½ small	1 small	1½ small	2 small	2½ small
Medium (1 oz)	-	½ medium	1 medium	1½ medium	2 medium
Large (2 oz)	-	-	-	½ large	½ large
Boston brown-bread, canned	-	½ slice	¾ slice	1 slice	1 slice
Bread-Pita Pocket	-	½ pocket	½ pocket	1 pocket	1 pocket
Bread-raisin, regular, sliced	-	½ slice	1 slice	1 ½ slices	2 slices
Bread-sandwich					
Regular, sliced	-	½ slice	1 slice	1½ slices	2 slices
Light, sliced	½ slice	1 slice	2 slices	2½ slices	3 slices
Breadstick					
Sesame-Keebler	2 sticks	4 sticks	5 sticks	7 sticks	9 sticks
Soft-Pillsbury	-	½ stick	¾ stick	1 stick	1½ sticks
Bun-hamburger or hotdog					
Regular	-	½ bun	½ bun	1 bun	1 bun
Light	-	½ bun	1 bun	1½ buns	1½ bun
Couscous-cooked	-	¼ cup	⅓ cup	½ cup	scant ⅔ cup
Crackers Saltine, club, Ritz, melba	2 regular	4 regular	6 regular	10 regular	12 regular
Crackers Oyster type	10 crackers	20 crackers	25 crackers	35 crackers	45 crackers
Crackers Triscuits	1 crackers	3 crackers	5 crackers	6 crackers	8 crackers
Crackers Sociables, Nabisco,	3 crackers	6 crackers	10 crackers	12 crackers	15 crackers
Crackers Wasa, Sesame Rye	2 pieces	5 pieces	7 pieces	10 pieces	12 pieces
Crackers, NIPS	8 Nips	15 Nips	25 Nips	30 Nips	40 Nips
Flours					
Cornmeal-whole grain	-	2 Tbsp	3 Tbsp	4 Tbsp	5 Tbsp
Oat Bran-raw	-	4 Tbsp	5 Tbsp	6 Tbsp	8 Tbsp
Rice flour-brown	-	1 Tbsp	2 Tbsp	2 Tbsp	3 Tbsp
Rye flour	-	2 Tbsp	3 Tbsp	4 Tbsp	5 Tbsp
Soy flour-roasted full fat	scant ¼ cup	⅓ cup	½ cup	⅔ cup	1 cup
Wheat germ	⅛ cup	¼ cup	⅓ cup	½ cup	scant ⅔ cup
White flour	-	2 Tbsp	3 Tbsp	4 Tbsp	5 Tbsp
Whole wheat	-	2 Tbsp	3 Tbsp	4 Tbsp	5 Tbsp

Effective Carbohydrate Content of Bread, Cereals, and Grains

Food	5 Grams	10 Grams	15 Grams	20 Grams	25 Grams
Grain cakes *	½ cake	1 cake	2 cakes	3 cakes	3 cakes
Melba toast	2 pieces	5 pieces	7 pieces	10 pieces	12 pieces
Muffin					
English, plain	-	-	½ muffin	¾ muffin	1 muffin
Corn, small	-	½ muffin	¾ muffin	1 muffin	1 muffin
Oat bran, mix					
Estee	-	½ muffin	1 muffin	1 muffin	1½ muffins
General Mills	-	-	½ muffin	¾ muffin	1 muffin
Oatmeal	-	-	scant ½ cup	½ cup	⅔ cup
Pancake-4"	-	½ cake	1 cake	1½ cakes	2 cakes
Pasta-cooked					
Egg noodles, spaghetti, macaroni	-	¼ cup	⅓ cup	½ cup	¾ cup
Chow mein noodles	-	⅓ cup	½ cup	¾ cup	1 cup
Noodles with rice-LaChoy	-	¼ cup	⅓ cup	½ cup	¾ cup
Lasagne-dry, uncooked	-	½ ounce	⅔ ounce	1 ounce	1¼ ounces
Piecrust-prepared-9"	-	-	⅛ crust	1/6 crust	1/5 crust
Pizza crust-small Thin-crust, 9"	-	-	⅛ crust	1/6 crust	1/5 crust
Popovers-small homemade	½ small	1 small	1½ small	2 small	2 small
Rice-cooked					
Brown	⅛ cup	¼ cup	⅓ cup	½ cup	scant ⅔ cup
White-long grain	⅛ cup	¼ cup	⅓ cup	½ cup	scant ⅔ cup
Wild	⅛ cup	¼ cup	scant ½ cup	½ cup	scant ¾ cup
Rice-fried	⅛ cup	¼ cup	⅓ cup	½ cup	½ cup
Risotto-cooked	-	⅛ cup	¼ cup	⅓ cup	½ cup
Rolls					
Crescent, small	½ roll	1 roll	1 roll	1½ rolls	2 rolls
Dinner	-	½ roll	1 roll	1½ rolls	1½ rolls
Stuffing, bread or corn bread	-	¼ cup	⅓ cup	½ cup	½ cup
Tortillas					
Corn-tostada, small taco shell	-	1 shell	2 shells	3 shells	3 shells
Flour-small	-	½ small	1 small	1 small	1½ small
Waffle-plain					
7" Diameter	-	-	½ waffle	¾ waffle	1 waffle
Frozen, small	-	½ waffle	1 waffle	1½ waffles	1½ waffles

*Grain cakes-pressed: Rice, oats, wheat popcorn, sesame, barley

Effective Carbohydrate Content of Vegetables

Food	5 Grams	10 Grams	15 Grams	20 Grams	25 Grams
Amaranth-boiled	1 cup	2 cups	Unlimited	Unlimited	Unlimited
Artichoke-boiled	-	½ medium	1 medium	1½ medium	2 medium
Artichoke hearts					
Boiled	¼ cup	½ cup	¾ cup	1 cup	1½ cups
Boiled, marinated in oil	¼ cup	½ cup	1 cup	1½ cups	1¾ cups
Arugula-raw	Unlimited	Unlimited	Unlimited	Unlimited	Unlimited
Asparagus					
Boiled	10 spears	20 spears	30 spears	Unlimited	Unlimited
Canned	1 cup	1½ cups	2½ cups	3 cups	4 cups
Frozen, boiled	6 spears	13 spears	20 spears	Unlimited	Unlimited
Bamboo shoots					
Raw	1 cup	2 cups	3 cups	5 cups	6 cups
Canned	1 cup	2 cups	3 cups	Unlimited	Unlimited
Bean salad-canned Pillsbury	⅛ cup	¼ cup	½ cup	⅔ cup	¾ cup
Beans					
Chili-Hunt's	scant ¼ cup	⅓ cup	½ cup	¾ cup	1 cup
Caliente-Joan of Arc	¼ cup	½ cup	⅔ cup	¾ cup	1 cup
Pork-Joan or Ark	⅛ cup	¼ cup	⅓ cup	½ cup	⅔ cup
Beans-refried	⅛ cup	⅓ cup	½ cup	⅔ cup	¾ cup
Beet greens-boiled	⅔ cup	1 cup	2 cups	2½ cups	3 cups
Beets					
Boiled, sliced	½ cup	¾ cup	1 cup	1½ cups	2 cups
Harvard, canned	-	¼ cup	⅓ cup	⅓ cup	½ cup
Pickled, canned	⅛ cup	¼ cup	⅓ cup	½ cup	⅔ cup
Black Beans	⅛ cup	¼ cup	⅓ cup	½ cup	¾ cup
Black turtle beans-canned	⅛ cup	¼ cup	⅓ cup	½ cup	⅔ cup
Broccoli					
Raw, chopped	2 cups	Unlimited	Unlimited	Unlimited	Unlimited
Boiled, chopped	1 cup	2 cups	3 cups	5 cups	Unlimited
Frozen, chopped	¾ cup	1½ cups	2½ cups	3 cups	4 cups
Broccoli/carrots frozen	¾ cup	1½ cups	2 cups	3 cups	4 cups
Broccoli/cauliflower frozen	1 cup	2 cups	2½ cups	3 cups	4 cups
Broccoli/corn/red pepper, frozen	⅓ cup	⅔ cup	1 cup	1⅓ cups	1½ cups
Broccoli/peppers/ bamboo shoots/ mushrooms	1 cup	2 cups	4 cups	5 cups	6 cups
Broccoli/pearl onions/red peppers, frozen	1 cup	2 cups	4 cups	5 cups	6 cups

Effective Carbohydrate Content of Vegetables

Food	5 Grams	10 Grams	15 Grams	20 Grams	25 Grams
Brussels Sprouts					
Boiled	5 sprouts	11 sprouts	15 sprouts	17 sprouts	25 sprouts
Butter Beans-canned	-	⅓ cup	½ cup	⅔ cup	1 cup
Cabbage-Chinese bok choy, raw	3 cups	Unlimited	Unlimited	Unlimited	Unlimited
Cabbage-green/red					
Raw	1½ cups	2 cups	5 cups	6 cups	Unlimited
Boiled	1½ cups	2 cups	3 cups	5 cups	6 cups
Carrots					
Raw	1 medium	2 medium	3 medium	4 medium	5 medium
Boiled, sliced	-	½ cup	1 cup	1½ cups	2 cups
Canned, sliced	¾ cup	1½ cups	2 cups	3 cups	4 cups
Frozen, sliced	½ cup	1 cup	1½ cups	2 cups	2½ cups
Cauliflower-raw, boiled, frozen	2 cups	4 cups	5 cups	Unlimited	Unlimited
Celery					
Raw	4 stalks	Unlimited	Unlimited	Unlimited	Unlimited
Boiled, diced	¾ cup	1½ cups	2 cups	3 cups	4 cups
Chard-Swiss-boiled	¾ cup	1 cup	2 cups	2½ cups	3 cups
Chickpeas					
Boiled	-	¼ cup	⅓ cup	½ cup	⅔ cup
Hummus	-	-	¼ cup	⅓ cup	½ cup
Chives-raw	Unlimited	Unlimited	Unlimited	Unlimited	Unlimited
Coleslaw	⅓ cup	½ cup	1 cup	1⅓ cup	1⅔ cups
Collard greens					
Boiled, chopped	½ cup	1 cup	2 cups	2½ cups	3 cups
Frozen, chopped	⅓ cup	¾ cup	1 cup	1½ cups	2 cups
Corn-white	-	¼ cup	⅓ cup	½ cup	¾ cup
Corn-yellow					
Boiled	-	¼ cup	⅓ cup	½ cup	⅔ cup
Frozen, boiled	-	⅓ cup	½ cup	⅔ cup	¾ cup
On the Cob	-	-	½ ear	½ ear	1 ear
Cowpeas (Black-eyed peas)					
Canned	-	⅓ cup	⅓ cup	½ cup	⅔ cup
Frozen, boiled	-	¼ cup	⅓ cup	½ cup	⅔ cup
Cucumber-raw	½ medium	1 medium	2 medium	3 medium	4 medium
Dandelion greens					
Raw	1 cup	2 cups	3 cups	4 cups	5 cups
Boiled, chopped	½ cup	1 cup	2 cups	3 cups	4 cups
Eggplant					
Raw	1 cup	2 cups	3 cups	4 cups	5 cups
Steamed, pieces	½ cup	1 cup	2 cups	3 cups	4 cups
Endive-raw	2 cups	4 cups	Unlimited	Unlimited	Unlimited
Fennel-fresh	¾ cup	1 cup	2 cups	3 cups	4 cups

Effective Carbohydrate Content of Vegetables

Food	5 Grams	10 Grams	15 Grams	20 Grams	25 Grams
Garlic	3 cloves	Unlimited	Unlimited	Unlimited	Unlimited
Ginger-raw, sliced	¼ cup	½ cup	Unlimited	Unlimited	Unlimited
Green Beans					
Boiled	½ cup	1 cup	2 cups	2½ cups	3 cups
Canned	1 cup	2 cups	3 cups	4 cups	5 cups
Frozen, whole	½ cup	1 cup	1½ cups	2 cups	3 cups
Hominy-canned	-	¼ cup	½ cup	⅔ cup	¾ cup
Italian-style veg-gies Frozen	⅓ cup	½ cup	⅔ cup	¾ cup	1 cup
Japanese-style veggies, frozen	⅓ cup	½ cup	¾ cup	1 cup	1¼ cups
Kale-boiled	½ cup	1 cup	2 cups	2½ cups	3 cups
Kelp-raw	¼ cup	½ cup	⅔ cup	¾ cup	2 cups
Kidney beans, red					
Boiled	-	¼ cup	⅓ cup	½ cup	⅔ cup
Canned	⅛ cup	¼ cup	⅓ cup	½ cup	⅔ cup
Leeks-boiled	½ cup	1 cup	1½ cups	2 cups	3 cups
Lentils-boiled	-	¼ cup	⅓ cup	½ cup	¾ cup
Lettuce					
Iceburg	Unlimited	Unlimited	Unlimited	Unlimited	Unlimited
Romaine	Unlimited	Unlimited	Unlimited	Unlimited	Unlimited
Lima Beans					
Boiled	⅛ cup	⅓ cup	½ cup	¾ cup	1 cup
Canned	⅛ cup	¼ cup	⅓ cup	½ cup	⅔ cup
Mushrooms					
Raw, pieces	1 cup	Unlimited	Unlimited	Unlimited	Unlimited
Steamed, canned	1 cup	2 cups	3 cups	4 cups	5 cups
Straw-canned	1 cup	Unlimited	Unlimited	Unlimited	Unlimited
Shiitake					
Whole, boiled	2 whole	4 whole	5 whole	8 whole	Unlimited
Whole, dried	2 whole	3 whole	5 whole	7 whole	8 whole
Mustard Greens					
Boiled, fresh	1½ cups	3 cups	Unlimited	Unlimited	Unlimited
Boiled, frozen	1 cup	2 cups	3 cups	4 cups	Unlimited
Navy Beans					
Boiled	-	¼ cup	⅓ cup	¾ cup	⅔ cup
Canned	-	-	¼ cup	½ cup	½ cup
Okra					
Boiled, slices	½ cup	¾ cup	1 cup	1½ cup	2 cups
Frozen, slices	⅓ cup	½ cup	1 cup	1⅓ cup	1½ cups
Onions					
Raw, chopped	½ cup	¾ cup	1 cup	Unlimited	Unlimited
Boiled, chopped	¼ cup	½ cup	¾ cup	1 cup	1¼ cups
Dehydrated	⅛ cup	¼ cup	⅓ cup	⅓ cup	½ cup
Onion, green, raw	1 cup	Unlimited	Unlimited	Unlimited	Unlimited
Parsley, raw	Unlimited	Unlimited	Unlimited	Unlimited	Unlimited

Effective Carbohydrate Content of Vegetables

Food	5 Grams	10 Grams	15 Grams	20 Grams	25 Grams
Parsnips, boiled	-	⅓ cup	½ cup	⅔ cup	1 cup
Peas-green					
Boiled	¼ cup	½ cup	¾ cup	1 cup	1¼ cups
Canned	⅓ cup	½ cup	1 cup	1⅓ cups	1½ cups
Peas-split, boiled	-	¼ cup	⅓ cup	½ cup	½ cup
Peas-sweet, can	¼ cup	½ cup	¾ cup	1 cup	1½ cups
Peppers-hot chili					
Raw	1 whole	2 whole	3 whole	4 whole	6 whole
Canned, chopped	½ cup	1 cup	1¾ cups	2 cups	Unlimited
Peppers-jalapeno, canned	½ cup	1 cup	Unlimited	Unlimited	Unlimited
Peppers-sweet					
Raw, chopped	1 cup	2 cups	Unlimited	Unlimited	Unlimited
Freeze-dried	1 cup	Unlimited	Unlimited	Unlimited	Unlimited
Peppers-sweet, yellow, raw	½ large	¾ large	1 large	1¾ large	2 large
Pimientos-canned	Unlimited	Unlimited	Unlimited	Unlimited	Unlimited
Pinto beans					
Boiled	⅛ cup	¼ cup	⅓ cup	½ cup	⅔ cup
Canned	⅛ cup	¼ cup	⅓ cup	½ cup	⅔ cup
Picante Style	⅛ cup	⅓ cup	½ cup	⅔ cup	¾ cup
Potato-sweet					
Baked, with skin	-	¼ medium	½ medium	¾ medium	1 medium
Boiled, mashed	-	-	-	¼ cup	⅓ cup
Potato-white					
Baked, with skin	-	-	¼ medium	⅓ medium	½ medium
Baked, no skin	-	¼ medium	⅓ medium	½ medium	¾ medium
Boiled, no skin	-	¼ medium	½ medium	⅔ medium	1 medium
Potato-new, whole, canned	-	⅓ cup	½ cup	⅔ medium	¾ medium
Potatoes-French fried	-	5	7	10	12
Potatoes-white, mashed	-	¼ cup	½ cup	⅔ cup	¾ cup
Pumpkin					
Boiled, mashed	¼ cup	½ cup	1 cup	1½ cups	2 cups
Canned, solid	¼ cup	½ cup	1 cup	1½ cups	2 cups
Radicchio-raw	Unlimited	Unlimited	Unlimited	Unlimited	Unlimited
Radishes					
Red, raw	Unlimited	Unlimited	Unlimited	Unlimited	Unlimited
White-raw, sliced	Unlimited	Unlimited	Unlimited	Unlimited	Unlimited

Effective Carbohydrate Content of Vegetables

Food	5 Grams	10 Grams	15 Grams	20 Grams	25 Grams
Red beans-canned	-	⅓ cup	½ cup	⅔ cup	1 cup
Rhubard-boiled	½ cup	1 cup	2 cups	3 cups	3½ cups
Rutabaga-boiled	⅓ cup	½ cup	1 cup	1½ cups	1¾ cups
Sauerkraut-canned	½ cup	¾ cup	1 cup	2 cups	2½ cups
Shallots-raw	3 Tbsp	Unlimited	Unlimited	Unlimited	Unlimited
Spinach					
Raw, chopped	Unlimited	Unlimited	Unlimited	Unlimited	Unlimited
Frozen, boiled	1 cup	3 cups	5 cups	Unlimited	Unlimited
Canned	3 cups	Unlimited	Unlimited	Unlimited	Unlimited
Squash-summer					
Raw, pieces	1 cup	2 cups	4 cups	5 cups	6 cups
Boiled	1 cup	2 cups	3 cups	4 cups	5 cups
Squash-winter					
Raw, pieces	½ cup	1 cup	1½ cups	2 cups	2½ cups
Boiled	⅓ cup	⅔ cup	1 cup	1½ cups	2 cups
Squash-spaghetti, baked or boiled	½ cup	1 cup	1½ cups	2 cups	2½ cups
Succotash					
Boiled	-	-	¼ cup	⅓ cup	½ cup
Canned/frozen	-	¼ cup	⅓ cup	½ cup	¾ cup
Tomatillo-raw	2 medium	5 medium	7 medium	10 medium	12 medium
Tomato					
Green, raw	1 medium	2 medium	3 medium	5 medium	6 medium
Red, raw	1 medium	2 medium	3 medium	5 medium	6 medium
Red, canned	½ cup	1 cup	1½ cups	2 cups	2½ cups
Red, with green chilies, canned	½ cup	1 cup	1½ cups	2 cups	2½ cups
Sun-dried	⅛ cup	¼ cup	½ cup	⅔ cup	¾ cup
Turnips-boiled	1 cup	2 cups	3 cups	4 cups	5 cups
Turnip greens					
Boiled, chopped	2 cups	4 cups	Unlimited	Unlimited	Unlimited
Canned, chopped	2 cups	3 cups	5 cups	Unlimited	Unlimited
Water chestnuts					
Raw, sliced	⅛ cup	¼ cup	½ cup	⅔ cup	¾ cup
Canned, whole	5 whole	10 whole	15 whole	Unlimited	Unlimited
Canned, sliced	¼ cup	½ cup	¾ cup	1 cup	1½ cups
White beans					
Boiled	-	¼ cup	⅓ cup	⅓ cup	½ cup
Canned	-	⅛ cup	¼ cup	⅓ cup	⅓ cup
Yams-baked or boiled, pieces	-	¼ cup	⅓ cup	½ cup	⅔ cup

Carbohydrate Bargains Under 1 Gram of Carbohydrate

1 cup alfalfa sprouts (0.4)
1 cup sliced bok choy (0.8)
1 tablespoon minced chives (0.1)
1 cup shredded lettuce (0.4)
½ cup sliced raw radicchio (0.9)
1 cup fresh spinach (0.6)
½ cup arugula (0.4)
1 celery rib (0.9)
½ cup sliced endive (0.8)
1 tbs chopped canned pimiento (0.6)
5 radishes (0.8)

Carbohydrate Bargains of 3 or Fewer Grams of Carbohydrate

¼ cup blackberries (2.9)
6 fresh asparagus spears (2.4)
½ cup canned asparagus (2.8)
4 frozen asparagus spears (2.9)
½ cup canned bamboo shoots (2.3)
1 cup chopped raw broccoli (2.2)
½ cup frozen broccoli/cauliflower florets (2.7)
¾ cup frozen broccoli/pearl onions/red peppers (2.6)
¼ cup cooked sliced carrots (3.0)
1 cup cauliflower florets (2.6)
½ medium cucumber (3)
¼ cup chopped leeks (2)
½ cup raw mushroom pieces (1.1)
½ cup cooked mushroom pieces (2.3)
5 whole enoki mushrooms (2)
½ cup chopped raw scallions (2.5)
½ cup chopped parsley (1.9)
½ cup chopped sweet pepper (2.4)
1 tablespoon chopped raw shallot (1.7)
½ cup boiled sliced summer squash (2.6)
1 medium tomatillo (2)
1 cup raw turnip greens (1.8) (or ½ cup cooked)

Carbohydrate Bargains of 5 or Fewer Grams of Carbohydrate

½ medium avocado (3.7)
¼ cup blueberries (4.3)
½ cup strawberries (3.3)
½ cup beet greens (3.9)
½ cup frozen Pillsbury broccoli/carrots (3.1)
4 brussels sprouts (3.4)
1 cup red or green cabbage (3.6)
1 medium carrot (5)
½ cup chopped Swiss chard (3.6)
½ cup chopped dandelion greens (3.3)
½ cup diced eggplant (3/2)
½ cup chopped fresh fennel (3.1)
½ cup sliced snap beans (3.8)
¼ cup frozen Japanese-style vegetables (3.7)
1 cup mustard greens (4)
1 whole hot chili pepper (4.3)
½ cup chopped jalapeno peppers (4.2)
½ cup boiled unsweetened rhubarb (3.5)
1 cup frozen spinach (3.1)
½ cup spaghetti squash (5)
1 cup raw diced summer squash (4)
1 medium tomato (4.3)
1 cup boiled turnip pieces (4.4)
4 whole water chestnuts (4)
½ cup canned sliced water chestnuts (4.5)
½ cup sliced wax beans (4.5)

Dr. Clark's Controlled Carbohydrate Diet *"Simplified"*

At CFWLS, everyone's diet will be individualized for them depending on their body composition, medical problems and long term goals. However, the *best way to begin* is to start watching your carbohydrate intake. Regulating your carbohydrate content has the greatest impact on fat storage since it is carbohydrate that directly stimulates the hormones **most** responsible for fat storage. So...if you are going to "count" something as you start your weight loss journey, it should be to count your carbohydrate intake.

Minimize your intake of:

Starches:

- Potato
- Rice
- Pasta
- Bread

Crumbly Carbohydrates (also referred to by Dr. Clark as the 6 C's):

- Chips
- Cookies
- Crackers
- Cereal
- Cake
- Candy

If you **MUST** have them:

- Use **very** limited portions
- Make sure they are whole grain

***Watch your fruit intake. Fruits tend to be high in sugar (sugar = carbohydrate).**

Foods of High Protein Content (Also Read Food Labels)

Food/Beverage	Serving Size	Protein	Calories	Carbs
MEAT, FISH, POULTRY				
Ground Sirloin (90% Lean)	3 oz	24.0 gm	195	0 gm
Roast	3 oz	19.0 gm	200	0 gm
Pork Tenderloin	3 oz	24.0 gm	147	0 gm
Pork Chop (lean)	3 oz	21.0 gm	184	0 gm
Duck	3 oz	21.0 gm	172	0 gm
Turkey Sausage	2 patties (2.4 oz)	13.0 gm	120	0 gm
Shrimp, boiled	3 oz	18.0 gm	85	0 gm
Tuna, in water	½ cup	28.0 gm	90	0 gm
Salmon	3 oz	21.0 gm	127	0 gm
Tilapia	3.5 oz	20.0 gm	96	0 gm
Flounder	3 oz	21.0 gm	99	0 gm
Lobster	1 cup	19.5 gm	85	0 gm
Scallops	3 oz	14.0 gm	75	0 gm
Baked Ham	3 oz	26.0 gm	130	0 gm
Chicken, dark	3.5 oz	30.0 gm	175	0 gm
Chicken, White	3.5 oz	33.0 gm	160	0 gm
Turkey Deli Meat	3 slices (3.5" square)	11.0	66	0 gm
Beef Jerky	1 oz	9.0 gm	116	3-10 gm
Peanut Butter	2 tbsp	8.0 gm	190	7 gm
Soy Nuts	1 oz	11.0 gm	128	9 gm
Almonds	1 oz	6.0 gm	169	6 gm
STARCHES				
Edamame (soy beans)	¼ cup	14.0 gm	130	12 gm
Fat free refried beans	½ cup	9.0 gm	135	22 gm
Pinto Beans	½ cup	7.0 gm	103	17 gm
Baked Beans	½ cup	8.0 gm	160	25 gm
Kidney Beans	½ cup	7.0 gm	110	18 gm
SOUPS				
Broth	½ cup	1.5 gm	25	0 gm
Low fat creamed Soup	1 cup	6.0-9.0 gm	90	15 gm
Chicken Noodle Soup	1 cup	4.0 gm	75	9 gm
Beans, Peas, or Lentil Soup	1 cup	7.5 gm	60	25 gm
Minestrone Soup	1 cup	5.0 gm	60	0 gm
MILK, CHEESE, YOGURT				
Cottage Cheese	½ cup	12.0 gm	80	6 gm
Skim mozzarella	1oz	6.0 gm	80	1 gm
Fat free Cheddar, Shredded	¼ cup	9.0 gm	35	0 gm
Skim Milk	1 cup/8 oz	8.0 gm	80	13 gm
Yogurt, light	1 cup	5.0-8.0 gm	60-90	6-12 gm
Egg, Large Size	1 egg	7.0 gm	75	1 gm
Egg Substitute	¼ cup	6.0 gm	30	0 gm
Tofu firm	3 oz	13.0 gm	117	4 gm

1 oz = 2 tablespoons 2oz = ¼ cup 3 oz = 1/3 cup 4 oz = ½ cup 8 oz = 1 cup

For More Recipes, Ideas, and great weight loss tips:

Check our blog for weekly recipes! Subscribe to the feed at:
www.cfwls.com/blog/

Pinterest	pinterest.com/cfwlsva/
Tumblr	cfwls.tumblr.com
Facebook	facebook.com/weightlossdrclark
Instagram	instagram.com/cfwls
Google+	plus.google.com/+CenterForWeightLossSuccessNewportNews
Linked In	linkedin.com/company/dr-clark's-center-for-weight-loss-success
Twitter	twitter.com/docweiightloss

Take advantage of these resources to help you stay on track

- **Free weekly podcasts** by Dr. Clark and other healthcare experts along with many of our own superstars – www.cfwls.com/podcasts
- Track your success and access us easily on our **portable App** – just search in the App Center for Center for Weight Loss Success on your portable devices such as iPhone, Android phone, iPod and iPad.
- **Losing Weight USA** – Get access to Dr. Clark every week. Details at www.LosingWeightUSA.com
- **Individualized Nutritional Counseling Sessions** – for accountability and I nformation to help you conquer your "problem habits" that may prevent you from ultimate success. These sessions are available individually or as a package of 6. Visit www.cfwls.com for more details.
- **My Weight Loss Academy** – 6 month digital program that also includes a 21-day Weight Loss Challenge for more quick results – also includes cool bonuses – visit www.MyWeightLossAcademy.com for details
- **Weight Management University™** - 6 month online and on-site weight loss program – visit http://cfwls.com/non-surgical-weight-loss/weight-management-university/ for details
- **Weight Loss Surgery** - with the most experience bariatric surgeon in the region along with our exclusive 12 month Weight Management University for Weight Loss Surgery™ program – visit http://cfwls.com/weight-loss-surgery/free-online-weight-loss-surgery-seminar/ to get started
- **Bio-Identical Hormone Replacement Therapy** – visit www.CenterforHormoneHealthandWellness.com for details

Printed in Dunstable, United Kingdom

91228666R00025